Intuitive Communication With Your Baby's Soul

Sandra K. Jones-Keller

For information about this book or personal one-on-one coaching, contact the author at: SandraJonesKeller.com

Intuitive Communication With Your Baby's Soul.

Cover Design: Thomas Keller, thomaskellerart.com

ISBN 978-1530298631

Dedication

This book is dedicated to all
the babies coming to Earth to
do great things!

CONTENTS

ACKNOWLEDGEMENTS

I wish to acknowledge my amazing husband, Thomas Keller, for his unwavering love and support of me. He challenges me to laugh at myself and the crazy, unexpected direction my life has taken. His artistry brought together my vision for the cover art in a way that's truly magical. Thomas, you are the best baby's daddy I could ask for!

Without my delightful and loving daughter, Mecca, I wouldn't be doing the work I'm doing now. I cherish each day I spend with her and am so grateful for the partnership we created while she was in utero.

A special thanks to my parents, Oscar and Ruthie Jones, for teaching me how to love and care for people and their unyielding acceptance of me. Mom and Dad, I hope I do you proud.

Deep thanks to Alison Blanco for taking time out of her very busy schedule to edit my book. I appreciate her keen eye and notes.

A heartfelt thank you to my friends, mentors and teachers who have taught and encouraged me on my spiritual journey throughout the years: Doreene Hamilton, Jill Courtenay, Louretta

Walker, Rev. Lynne Herod-Deverges, and Dr. Carolyne "Isis" Fuqua.

Sweet hugs to Wendi Cartwright-Eckstein for letting me sit by her pool to veg while I was pregnant; girl, you helped me get through some rough patches.

A profound thank you to Evelyn Thompson for being my pregnancy coach, practitioner, dear friend and confidant. Evie, you walked with me through the biggest challenge I've ever faced. You held the truth of my wholeness and oneness throughout it all and I am eternally grateful!

Lastly, thank you to all the moms, dads and grandparents who have shared their baby communication stories with me. Your experiences inspire others to go beyond the norm.

INTRODUCTION

They say that whenever you schedule an appointment for a spiritual reading or healing energy session, the work begins the minute you make the commitment. That's because you have just sent a signal to the universe saying, "I am ready for a change. I am ready for a healing. I am open and willing." You see, you are always surrounded and supported by divine beings who love and honor you. But until you ask for their help, they wait patiently, for they cannot and will not interfere with your free will. You must invite them in.

The same is true with this book. Simply by finding it and opening it you have set a new course of possibility for your relationship with your unborn or newborn baby. Maybe you prayed for guidance, maybe a friend recommended it to you, or better yet, maybe your baby sent it your way. Either way, the constructs of reality are shifting and you have stepped into a new paradigm of being. All of the information I present may not resonate with you, but trust that you will receive whatever it is you need to receive from this book, at the time that is right for you. There is no mistake that we are here together.

I view this book as validation of experiences   moms,   dads   and grandparents are already having with the babies that are coming into the physical Earth plane. One mom approached me after a workshop and thanked me for presenting this information. She said that when she was pregnant, her baby communicated with her, but she never told anyone because she feared being ostracized or thought crazy. Mothers have told me that they knew what their baby would look like before it was born, or knew things about it from communicating with it in utero. Intuitive two-way communication with an unborn baby is not new, it just hasn't been talked about openly.

As an Intuitive Pregnancy Coach and Spiritual Energy Healer I teach new moms, pregnant moms and want to be moms how to develop intuitive two-way communication with their unborn and newborn babies. I use a purely spiritual approach to pregnancy and trying to conceive.

Think of me as your anchor and guide to lean on when you feel no one understands what you're going through. I teach you the same tools and principles I used when I was pregnant. Even though I had been on my own spiritual journey for over a decade at the time of my high-risk pregnancy, I still needed someone to call to keep me grounded and sane. It's okay to need and ask for help.

My approach is gentle and loving. I've been scared, frustrated and uncertain just like you may be. In order to support you during this important rite of passage, I've taken my knowledge and experience and created processes to help you find balance, peace and empowerment! The tools outlined in this book can assist you with tapping into the Universal Power that is available each and every moment of the day.

During a spiritual energy healing session with a client, I never know what's going to be revealed: I've had the spirits of miscarried babies come through to explain why they have changed their minds about being born;

I've had unborn souls clarify what they need from their parents in order to incarnate; and I've had babies tell me they're fine. As you can see, a spiritual reading can be quite elucidating!

One thing you may notice in this book is I often refer to an unborn baby's soul/spirit as "it" instead of the traditional pronouns "he" or "she", "him" or "her". Please don't take offense. I do this not out of disrespect, but because there is no gender in spirit. It is not until we incarnate into a physical body that we become a male or female. Additionally, throughout our incarnations, we have been men and women, different races and creeds, rich and poor, benevolent and tyrannical. So my reference of "it" in no way diminishes the magnitude of the human spirit and the journeys it has taken!

My objective for you is that at the end of this book you will have the tools and confidence to establish intuitive two-way communication with your baby. It may not happen overnight, but with patience and practice you can develop a deep spiritual bond with your child that will last a lifetime. You are not just having a baby, you are fulfilling a spiritual contract!

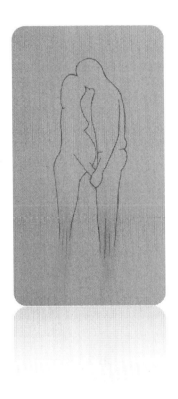

"I am strong and healthy. My baby is well."

Notes:

CHAPTER 1

THE SET UP

MY STORY

At 41 years old, I became pregnant with my daughter Mecca. Before I even went to the doctor, I knew something was off. I was only a few days late with my cycle, but I looked like I was 3-4 months pregnant. Turns out I had a couple of large fibroid tumors, one of which was at the base of my uterus. The doctor's prognosis for me was pretty dire: I'd be bedridden for most of my pregnancy, Mecca would be born 3 months premature, and I would have a C-section.

I did what I always do when confronted with a challenge or fear. I got busier and deeper into my spiritual practices. I began meditating more. I spent time in quiet contemplation and reflection. I did spiritual mind treatments (affirmative prayer) with a practitioner. I connected with nature, read my spiritual books, wrote out positive affirmations, and most of all, I listened deeply and intently to my intuition.

What ensued over the next 8 ½ months was a partnership between me and my unborn daughter to have a healthy and successful pregnancy. I did have a C-section, but I carried her full term. I was never bedridden. As a matter of fact, I worked part-time up until the weekend before she was born. And Mecca came home at the end of my hospital stay. How did I beat my prognosis? I developed intuitive two-way communication with my baby. I talked to my unborn daughter and she answered back! Yes, answered back!

THE FIRST TIME MECCA TALKED BACK TO ME

I was about three months pregnant the first time Mecca talked back to me. Thomas (my then boyfriend, now

3

husband) and I were at a spiritual conference in Las Vegas. We were scheduled to return to Los Angeles on Monday. What Thomas hadn't told me was that he had checked us out of our room on Sunday and we were going to spend the last night with his friend (to save some money.) Well I was pregnant and uncomfortable and very annoyed. I didn't want to share a room with someone else, so I told him I would catch a ride back to Los Angeles. He totally surprised me by asking, "Did you ask Mecca what she wants to do?"

My first thought was "Why do I need to ask her? It's my body, I get to decide." But I thought I would humor him. I went into meditation, quieted my mind and asked Mecca "Do you want to go home with me or stay in Vegas with Daddy?" Before I barely finished the question, I heard a voice in my mind say "I want to stay here with Daddy." Now this was not the answer I wanted! I had my own agenda, I wanted to go home and thought for sure that she would want to go with me. Not to be deterred, I asked her again—the same answer. I knew this was her voice because the answer wasn't what I wanted to hear. I went back to Thomas and begrudgingly said "We're staying."

HOW I CREATED A PARTNERSHIP WITH MECCA

After my first two-way telepathic (an internal voice I heard in my head) conversation with Mecca in Las Vegas, she and I had access to a deeper level of communication. Before this, I had been simply talking to her, rubbing my belly and loving her silently. Now I knew she could and would answer back!

I began to rely on her feedback and wisdom to support me during my pregnancy. I was quite emotional and often scared after several of my doctor's appointments. My doctor would say with complete confidence things like: "Mecca will be born early because your uterus can only stretch so far and you are pretty close to that maximum." Or "There's a chance your fibroids might

interfere with the growth of your baby."
At one point they couldn't find her
heartbeat after extensive searching. She
had carved a space for herself in
between my fibroids and was hanging
out there comfortably.

Almost daily I would ask Mecca how
she was doing. Her answer was always
the same, "I'm fine mom, take care of
yourself." I could feel her strong, loving,
confident energy ushering me along the
way. Because I knew she was fine, I had
the strength and determination to focus
on myself, doing what I needed to do to
carry her safely to full-term.

The most frightening part of the 38
weeks was the day of my delivery. I had

a scheduled C-section first thing in the morning. The staff tested and retested my blood. They delayed taking me into the operating room. I could feel the fear and apprehension all around me. I realized the doctors were afraid of excessive bleeding during my procedure. They were preparing for all possibilities. I consciously decided I was not going to bleed to death on the table. I literally left my body and went into a trance-like state holding the vibration of life, wellness and motherhood. It wasn't until I heard them say "she's all clear" that I took a deep breath and reentered my body. I have never had to be so focused and determined as I was in that moment. I concentrated on living and being with my daughter! I was completely connected to her and could feel her strength even through this distress.

A HIGHER POWER

What the doctors didn't know that I knew was that there was a higher power than the medical profession that I was calling on throughout my pregnancy and delivery. I call it God, some may call it Spirit, Holy Spirit, Allah, Christ, angels; you may call it whatever is comfortable for you. This Universal Power completely supported and guided me on this journey. My doctors and nurses had based their predictions on what they had seen in the past. Had I bought into the medical professional's experiences, then my original prognosis probably would have occurred. Fortunately, I had my spiritual toolbox to pull from which assisted me in creating a different reality than the predictions I had received.

After Mecca was born, I would check in with her telepathically to see if she had woken up if I was downstairs and she was upstairs, or ask her how she was feeling if she didn't look like her normal self. I still check in with her telepathically even after 10 years. I do this by getting quiet, closing my eyes, and focusing on reaching out to her higher self. I like to call it Mother's intuition stepped up!

Intuitive Communication With Your Baby's Soul

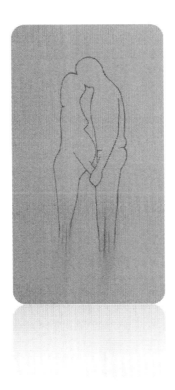

"I tap into my intuition easily and
effortlessly. I am open to receive
divine guidance."

Notes:

CHAPTER 2
THIS THING CALLED INTUITION

WHAT IS INTUITION?

Intuition is your sixth sense, your sense of knowing. It is that quiet, small voice within that can guide you and keep you out of trouble. Some people refer to it as a "gut feeling." Merriam-Webster's defines intuition as: "a natural ability or power that makes it possible to know something without any proof or evidence; a feeling that guides a person

15

to act a certain way without fully understanding why; something that is known or understood without proof or evidence." Intuition is a muscle that needs to be developed. The more you use it, the more you learn to recognize and trust it.

WHY IS INTUITION IMPORTANT NOW?

Tapping into your intuition is more important now than ever before! The consciousness of our planet is rising. We are being called to be more heart-centered than brain centered. It is through your heart that you feel love, compassion, justice, certainty, and wholeness. It is through your heart and third eye, the area located at the center of your forehead, that you feel your intuition; that you meld with your higher self, your spiritual wisdom. Connecting with your heart, third eye and higher self opens up access to communicating with your baby telepathically. You can learn to feel and hear its voice and connect with their soul. At this point in our evolutionary history, the time is ripe for intuitive, telepathic communication with our babies!

YOU ALREADY USE YOUR INTUITION

You have developed and trusted your five senses all of your life, now it's time to tap into your sixth sense. We all have and use our intuition on a regular basis. For example, maybe you are driving down the street and your inner voice tells you to turn right instead of left, and you find out later you avoided a major traffic jam by turning right. Or you have the random thought to call a friend and they say, "I was just thinking about you." You have tapped into your intuition!

Recently, a friend invited my daughter to go ice skating with her family on a

Sunday night. I trust this friend, but something inside of me said "not this time," and I declined the invitation. Turns out the ice skating rink was closed for a special event, and they drove all the way to the rink for nothing! At the time I didn't know why I said no, but I trusted my instincts and didn't let my daughter go. The bottom line is the more you use and follow your internal guidance, your intuition, the more confident and connected you will feel. I'm sure if you think about it, you've had similar experiences on multiple occasions.

EXERCISES TO DEVELOP YOUR INTUITION

As I've said before, intuition is a muscle that needs to be exercised and developed. Just like going to the gym, the more you "work out" your intuitive muscles, the stronger and more reliable they will become. You may wonder, "How do I start?" Here are a few easy exercises for you to practice developing your intuition. Take your time with them. Go at your own pace. This is not a race. There is no finish line.

1. Automatic writing: Sit down with your journal and a pen. Silently ask a question. It could be something that's been troubling

you for a while or something you need clarity on. Wait quietly for a response. Once your pen starts moving, don't stop until you're done. Let the information flow freely without reading it or analyzing it. You will be able to feel when you're done writing. Then you can read it. Take the information in without judgement. This is a great way to connect with your higher self and start your intuitive juices flowing.

2. Pillow question: Write down a question on a piece of paper. Put it under your pillow before you go to bed. Ask for the answer to be revealed to you during your

sleep. Before you get up in the morning sit quietly and write down any messages you received or any thoughts or feelings you have. You may not get the answer the first time out, but keep practicing. This is a great way to tap into your dreams and subconscious for answers.

3. Meditation: (Chapter 10 covers meditation if you are unfamiliar with the process.) Ask a question at the beginning of your meditation, and ask for a clear answer to be revealed to you. Let go of the question during your meditation and trust that it is being handled by your higher

self. Write down any thoughts or insights at the end of your meditation.

These are techniques I have used over the years to tap into my intuition. Practice the above mentioned and come up with your own. Play around with different ideas. There is no right way to develop your intuition. Each journey is very personal and distinct!

Notes

1. Intuition. 2016. In Merriam-Webster.com
    Retrieved January 26, 2016 from
    http://www.merriam-webster.com/dictionary/intuition

Intuitive Communication With Your Baby's Soul

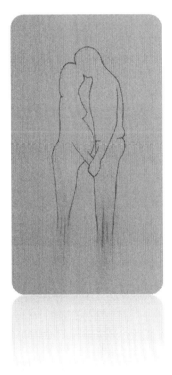

"I rejoice in this New Age of
wisdom and freedom."

Notes:

CHAPTER 3

WE ARE IN THE NEW AGE AND WHAT IT MEANS FOR YOU!

WHAT IS THE NEW AGE?

The term New Age has been floating around for decades. I remember listening to the song Aquarius/Let the Sunshine In by 5th Dimension when I was a kid back in the late 1960's. I loved the melody, but had no idea what the song actually meant. Fast forward to present day. I looked up the lyrics and smiled. Clues have been all around us foretelling the dynamic changes taking place on our planet and in our solar system. Here's just the first verse of the song:

> *When the moon is in the seventh*
> *house*
> *And Jupiter aligns with Mars*
> *And peace will guide the planets*
> *And love will steer the stars*
> *This is dawning of the Age of*
> *Aquarius*
> *Age of Aquarius.*
> *Aquarius, Aquarius.*

This song refers to the Precession of the Equinoxes which I'll discuss in the next section. It is referring to this New Age of now.

28

Many people may find the term New Age frightening because of all the negative things they've heard or read. I personally find this time exciting with all the new possibilities available; look, you are reading a book about communicating with your baby's soul!

In a live Kryon Channeling entitled, "Demystifying the New Age - 3 " by Lee Carol, an American channeler, speaker and author, this period is defined eloquently, "When we talk about New Age and esoteric beliefs, we use the terms interchangeably. The term New Age can often mean cult in certain cultures, so we often use esoteric instead. Both words mean a belief system that is unique on the

29

planet and has no structure or doctrine. It has no central book. It has no prophet to worship and there's no place where there is a central headquarters. There's no place to report to and there are no rules. There is no membership and no record of who started it. What a system! It's out of the perception of any logical, organized system, because it has no organization." He goes on to say, "There is a central core belief that God is inside; that souls come to the planet many times; and that humanity is part of a benevolent system creating the spiritual evolution of Earth."

I hope this explanation of the New Age provides some insight and clarity about this period of time on our planet. If you watch the news, there is a lot of darkness and negativity running amuck; plenty of reasons to be fearful. But rest assured, millions of people are focused on bringing in and being the light.

THE PRECESSION OF THE EQUINOXES

Over the past several years there have been many planetary changes that have been in the news. The most recognizable date was the winter solstice on December 21st, 2012, which was the end of the Mayan calendar. This event was the Precession of the Equinoxes, which was the end of an approximately 2,160 year cycle, moving us out of the Age of

Pisces into the Age of Aquarius. Basically, we are moving and have moved into the next Great Cycle.

Qualities of this New Age include love, freedom, peace and spiritual awareness among many others. The water bearer, which represents the zodiacal sign of Aquarius, is a symbol that we can now receive, understand and hold greater levels of wisdom and higher levels of consciousness. In the past, we relied on educators, ministers, trainers and such to teach us information. Now we can connect with our higher selves and our intuition to recognize the God within us.

This New Age has ushered in more light and love than ever before. Our intuition is keener, our energy fields are lighter, and we have the ability and capacity to connect with higher realms of consciousness. During this time, it is easier to connect with your unborn baby because of all the cosmic energy shifts that have occurred. You can now establish a deep spiritual bond and partnership with your baby before it's born!

LIFTING OF THE VEIL

I like to compare the planetary energy shifts that are occurring to a fog lifting. Imagine that you walk out your front door one morning and the fog is so thick you can't see your own car parked in the driveway or your neighbor's house across the street. Then the sun begins to shine and the fog burns off. You walk outside again, and sure enough, you can see your car and your neighbor's house. Did they ever go away, or were they just obstructed by the thick fog? They were obstructed, of course!

Each lunar and solar eclipse has great significance. Each sun flare, new moon and full moon over the past few years has been adding more light and divine energy to our planet. This light energy has been dissolving the fog (the veil that has kept us from seeing clearly.) With this light comes heightened awareness and keener intuition. You have the ability to be more open and conscious than ever before. Information is processed faster and understood at a deeper level. You are more in tune with your higher self. All of this contributes to your ability to develop a deep spiritual bond with your baby! It's your chance to create a lasting life-long partnership with your child now.

ATTRIBUTES OF THE NEW AGE KID

The children being born are definitely different from previous generations. Often times, I am in awe of my daughter, not just because she's mine, but because of her open heart, generosity, expression of joy, wisdom and her willingness to forgive. She knows things because she feels them intuitively. She's grounded and centered. She's clear and certain. She's kind and helpful.

As we continue to ascend in consciousness (release our negative baggage, open our hearts, love and have more compassion) we remember more and feel more. Our children come into this world with a higher capacity for awareness than we did. They are more connected to their higher selves. I love the following two stories that exhibit what I mean:

> One mom told me how her five month old son said a complete sentence. When she reacted with shock, the boy got a look on his

face that said "Oh, maybe I shouldn't have done that," and went back to simply making baby noises.

While I was editing this book, the Universe put me into a position to overhear a mother talking with her young daughter (two-three years old.)

Daughter, "Mom you're the best mom I've ever had!"

Mother, "I'm the only mother you've ever had."

Daughter, "No, I've <u>never</u> had this before!"

I knew what the daughter was trying to tell her mother, but I don't think her mother understood it. The daughter was telling her mother that in all of her previous lifetimes, she'd never had someone love and care for her in the ways her mother did. I felt the deep gratitude and fondness the daughter was expressing to her mother.

More and more of these types of incidents are taking place between parents and children. The New Age is upon us. We need to be ready to support our New Age kids in ways that anchor and encourage them, not try to fit them into a box or stifle their intuitive nature. They know what they know because they feel it and remember it from previous incarnations.

Notes

1. The 5th Dimension. "Aquarius/Let The Sunshine In."
    The Age of Aquarius.
    Soul City. 1969

2. Carol, Lee.
    "Demystifying the New Age - 3 ".
    Live Kryon Channeling
    Edmonton, AB, Canada. January 25, 2014
    https://www.kryon.com/CHAN2014/k_channel14_EDMONTON-14.html

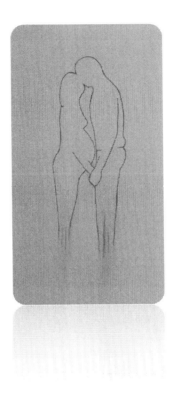

"I acknowledge my pregnancy as
a spiritual agreement."

Notes:

CHAPTER 4
LET'S START THINKING ABOUT PREGNANCY DIFFERENTLY

PREGNANCY ISN'T JUST ABOUT BIOLOGY

Having a baby isn't just about biology; it is a spiritual agreement! A baby is a conscious, sentient being. Conscious meaning aware of and responding to one's surroundings; awake. Sentience is the ability to feel, perceive or to experience. The fetus is the baby in your belly, but what animates it and gives it life is the spirit/soul waiting to come into the physical body. Without a spirit ready to come through, there is no baby. A great deal of soul planning takes place between a child, its parents and their higher selves before a spirit incarnates. Therefore, giving birth is not a random or chance occurrence. The child you're carrying has chosen you to be its parent, guardian and way-shower in this life. What a magnificent responsibility you've agreed to!

Keep in mind that children are not coming here for our benefit and pleasure. These spirits have their own

44

purposes and agendas for life. Many are coming to do great things here on Earth and they require the proper environment in which to incarnate! In a reading/healing energy session that I did for a couple trying to conceive, who already had multiple miscarriages, the spirit of the baby came in to explain why it hadn't incarnated yet. Some of the reasons included: the parents were extremely busy trying to get a new venture off the ground and didn't really have time for a new baby; there was dissention amongst the other children about a new baby coming into the family; and most of all, it didn't want to be controlled by the parents. Once the couple received this clarity, they began correcting the issues blocking the child from being born.

A child chooses his or her parents for the conditions it needs to fulfill its life lessons. There has to be a match in vibrations. Millions of women experience miscarriages each year. Most medical professionals believe miscarriages occur due to physical abnormalities like a chemical pregnancy or chromosomal abnormality. Very few consider the spiritual aspects of a miscarriage; possibly a miscarriage happens because the soul decides to release the body. It could be waiting for the right time or environment, or may not come through at all.

Before I met Thomas, I had been together with my first husband for 10 years, eight married, and two dating, and I never got pregnant. I was frustrated and disappointed. I desperately wanted to be a mother and thought my chances of having a baby ended with my marriage at 36 years old. Then Thomas came along, and I was pregnant within three months of us being in the same city, (we dated long distance for six months) despite my large fibroid tumors and my age. By the way, Thomas was 49 when I conceived so we were both considered older parents. In other words, my daughter incarnated when the timing and environment was right for her!

47

RELATIONSHIP BETWEEN A MEDIUM AND YOUR BABY

We are spiritual beings from the beginning to the end! Our spirit doesn't start at conception. It has existed and will continue to exist after its lifetime on Earth. That is why mediums, someone that can communicate with a deceased person, can connect with loved ones. They are connecting with the spirit of the person who is no longer physically here.

Let's circle this concept around. A baby is a spiritual being. Its spirit didn't just come into existence with your pregnancy. It is an eternal being. With this in mind, you can ask your baby directly what it needs to be best taken care of in this moment. If you have miscarried in the past, ask the spirit of the baby why it miscarried. Ask it if it's coming back. You can gain tremendous clarity and insight from this information. You don't need a medium to speak with your unborn baby! You can do it naturally given an openness and willingness, combined with practice and patience. Remember your child has chosen you to be its mother and is excited to be in contact with you!

VALUE OF CREATING A SPIRITUAL BOND WITH YOUR CHILD

Having telepathic conversations with your unborn or newborn baby gives you an unprecedented level of confidence and security. You are no longer relying on sources outside of yourself for validation and confirmation that you are on the right track. You know you are doing the best thing for your baby because the information comes straight from the source—your child!

In addition, a paradigm shift in parenting can occur once you create a spiritual bond with your little one. As you recognize your child as an intelligent being, and not just a baby, you intuitively treat them differently. Part of our pact as parents with these children is to help them navigate living on earth, to "show them the ropes." They are not our possessions, they do not need us to plan out their lives, worry about their futures, or live out our fantasies and agendas through them. They need us to be loving, encouraging, compassionate, supportive guardians for them on their own journey through life.

Intuitive Communication With Your Baby's Soul

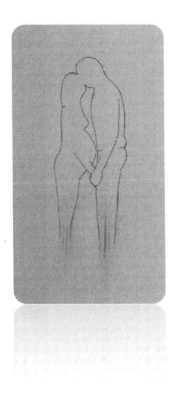

"I am grounded and centered."

<u>Notes:</u>

CHAPTER 5
GROUNDING IS AN IMPORTANT TOOL

WHAT IS GROUNDING?

A ship in the ocean drops its anchor to be grounded in one place. Otherwise it would drift back out to sea. You ground yourself to bring your own energy back into your body and energy field. At times, your energy gets scattered. You ground yourself to start thinking clearly, to receive divine guidance. You can't hear your intuition if you're scattered and frazzled. Grounding yourself gives you more access to communication with your higher self. Once you ground yourself, you can begin to communicate with your baby.

GROUNDING EXERCISE

- Sit in a chair with your feet flat on the floor.

- Clear everything from your lap. Have your palms up or down on your lap.

- Take three deep breaths. Relax your entire body.

- Picture in your mind's eye the area between your tail bone and pelvic region. (This is your first or root chakra. I will talk more about chakras in the next chapter.) You are going to ground this area to the center of the earth.

- Now you are going to create your grounding cord. Your grounding cord can be a big thick rope, or a tree trunk, or even a robust waterfall. Anything that feels solid and sturdy to you that will help you to feel anchored. Picture your grounding cord in your mind's eye.

- Picture a barbell in the middle of your root chakra.

- Wrap your grounding cord tightly around the barbell then shoot it down to the center of the earth.

- Find a huge rock or tree to attach the end of your grounding cord to then pull it tightly.

- You are now grounded.

- Relax into this experience.

********   .

For some of you this may be the first time you've ever really felt grounded or anchored into your body. You can do this several times per day, and it will help you to feel more peaceful and connected.

HOW DOES GROUNDING HELP YOU BOND WITH YOUR BABY?

You will start to notice the difference between being grounded and not grounded. I definitely feel more anchored and clear when I'm grounded. The first thing I always did before my doctor's appointments when I was pregnant was ground myself. Grounding helped me deal with all the feelings of fear and uncertainty and helped me to have a clear channel to my daughter. I was able to take a moment and feel the truth inside of me because I was grounded. Often times during my pregnancy I had to ground myself several times throughout the day since I would get caught up in the doctor's fearful predictions for me.

Ultimately grounding yourself and opening your chakras is the key to developing intuitive two-way communication with your baby. Both will assist you with accessing information from the higher realms in ways that are truly delightful!

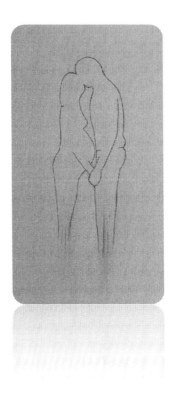

"My chakras are open. My energy flows freely."

<u>Notes:</u>

CHAPTER 6

CHAKRAS

WHAT IS A CHAKRA?

Chakra (pronounced sha-kra or cha-kra) is an energy center. It is a Sanskrit word that means wheel or disc. You have seven main chakras that run down the center of your body. You take in, release and process energy and information through your chakras.

When your chakras are open, energy moves easily, you are able to process information with less effort, and you move fluidly in the world. When your chakras are closed, you can feel blocked and stuck: you can feel disconnected from yourself, your loved ones and your life. You need open chakras to communicate with your baby and higher self and to develop your intuition.

YOU ALREADY EXPERIENCE YOUR CHAKRAS

You already experience open and closed chakras and you may not even know it! Let's talk about your heart chakra (fourth) and throat chakra (fifth) for a moment.

Have you ever fallen in love? Do you remember feeling like your heart was going to burst open? How do you feel when you think about your baby? Warm and fuzzy, huh? Or have you ever watched a movie and suddenly started crying because you were so moved by a scene? Well that's your heart chakra opening and responding to your environment. That's love pouring through you.

What about a closed chakra? Well, have you ever tried to say something and you just couldn't get the words out? Or maybe your throat suddenly felt tight or dry. Could be your fifth chakra is closed. When your throat chakra is closed, it's difficult to communicate clearly; to actually spit the words out. An open throat chakra supports you in your communication both verbally and nonverbally.

Deepak Chopra, a public speaker, author, and expert on alternative medicine and spirituality, says, "Each of the seven chakras are governed by spiritual laws, principles of consciousness that we can use to cultivate greater harmony, happiness, and well-being in our lives and in the world."

Actively practicing opening your chakras will get you in touch with your higher self on deeper levels than ever before. As you open your heart and mind to divine information you will be guided to what's best for you and your baby. You will open up your intuitive channels so that you can actually hear and commune with your baby.

THE SEVEN MAIN CHAKRAS

Chakras.info explains chakras this way, "Each chakra has its own vibrational frequency that is depicted through a specific chakra color, and governs specific functions that help make you, well, human." I love their following descriptions of the chakras:

First Chakra

- The root chakra is the first chakra. Its energy is based on the earth element. It's associated with the feeling of safety and grounding. It's at the base of the chakra system and lays the foundation for expansion in your life. The corresponding color for this chakra is red.

Second Chakra

- The sacral chakra is the second chakra. It is associated with the emotional body, sensuality, and creativity. Its element is water and as such, its energy is characterized by flow and flexibility. The function of the sacral chakra is directed by the principle of pleasure. The corresponding color for this chakra is orange.

Third Chakra

- The Solar Plexus chakra is the third chakra. It is associated with the expression of will, power, mental abilities, and personal responsibility. Its element is fire and as such, its energy is characterized by transmutation and heat. The Solar Plexus chakra is directed by the principle of power and the intellect. The corresponding color for this chakra is yellow.

Fourth Chakra

- The Heart chakra is the fourth chakra. Located at the center of the chakra system, it bridges the spiritual and the earthly chakras. It is associated with the many expressions of love, compassion, and relating to others and oneself. The function of the Heart chakra is driven by the principle of connection and integration. The corresponding color for this chakra is green.

Fifth Chakra

- The Throat chakra is the fifth chakra. Located at the center of the neck at the level of the throat, it is the passage of the energy between the lower parts of the body and the head. The function of the Throat chakra is driven by the principle of expression and communication. The corresponding color for this chakra is blue.

Sixth Chakra

- The third eye chakra is the sixth chakra. Located on the forehead, between the eyebrows, it is the center of intuition and foresight. The function of the third eye chakra is driven by the principle of openness and imagination. The corresponding color for this chakra is indigo.

Seventh Chakra

- The crown chakra is the seventh chakra. Located at the top of the head, it gives us access to higher states of consciousness as we open to what is beyond our personal preoccupations and visions. The function of the Crown chakra is driven by consciousness and gets us in touch with the universal. The corresponding colors for this chakra are white or violet.

As I said earlier, you need open chakras to communicate with your baby and higher self; to develop your intuition. In the next section, I will guide you through a meditation to ground your chakras and help you open up to intuitive communication with your baby.

Notes

1. Chopra, Deepak.
   Insights For Living. *What Everyone Needs To Know About Their Chakras*. (2013)
   http://www.mindbodygreen.com/0-11943/what-everyone-needs-to-know-about-their-chakras.html

2. Chakras A to Z Reference Guide For Beginners & Healers. *What Are The Chakras?* (2015)
   http://www.chakras.info/

3. Chakras A to Z Reference Guide For Beginners & Healers. *Introducing The 7 Major Chakras.* (2015) http://www.chakras.info/

.

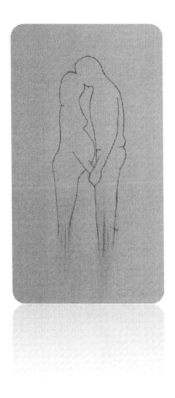

"I develop a deep connection with
my baby through meditation."

<u>Notes:</u>

CHAPTER 7

MEDITATION

WHAT IS MEDITATION?

There are a variety of definitions for meditation, but in its simplest form, to meditate means:

- to quiet your mind;

- to contemplate or reflect;

- to actively practice mindfulness (concentrating on your breath or by repeating a word or statement) to reach higher levels of awareness.

77

PURPOSE OF MEDITATION

Pregnancy and having a baby is an important rite of passage for a woman. It is also a time of extreme emotional and physical changes in the body. Learning to meditate will assist you in staying peaceful, joy-filled and confident! You will be better equipped to navigate all of the changes taking place in your body and life.

According to Deepak Chopra, "The real purpose of meditation isn't to tune out and get away from it all but to tune in and get in touch with your true Self – that eternal aspect of yourself that goes beyond all the ever-changing, external circumstances of your life. In meditation you dive below the mind's churning surface, which tends to be filled with repetitive thoughts about the past and worries about the future, into the still point of pure consciousness. In this state of transcendent awareness, you let go of all the stories you've been telling yourself about who you are, what is limiting you, and where you fall short – and you experience the truth that your deepest Self is infinite and unbounded."

TYPES OF MEDITATION

There are many different types of meditation. Some of the most popular as described by The Institute of Noetic Sciences are:

Concentrative Meditation

- In this practice the objective is to cultivate a single-pointed attention on some object, such as a sound, an image, the breath, or a flame. The most well-known and researched form of the concentrative type in the West is Transcendental Meditation (TM).

Open Awareness

- The objective of these forms of meditative practices is to open the mind into a panoramic awareness of whatever is happening without a specific focus.

Mindfulness

- The most popular, widely
  adapted, and widely researched
  meditation technique in the West.
  It is a combination of
  concentration and open
  awareness. The practitioner
  focuses on an object, such as the
  breath, bodily sensations,
  thoughts, feelings, or sounds.

Guided Meditation

- All forms of meditation can be
  guided, and many are often
  practiced with recorded or in-
  person guidance at first, and then
  later with decreasing need for
  explicit guidance. In one form,

called guided imagery, the practitioner follows auditory guidance from a teacher or recording that elicits certain images, affirmations, states (such as peacefulness), or imagined desired experiences.

IS MEDITATION NECESSARY TO COMMUNICATE WITH YOUR BABY?

Meditation will help still and quiet your mind so you can hear intuitive information. Meditation is a tool. Meditation helps you ground yourself. Meditation gives you access to more of yourself. It assists with developing your intuitive muscles which helps you hear your baby. So yes, I believe some form of meditation is necessary to develop intuitive two-way communication with your unborn or newborn baby! Just like everything else, meditation can be guided by your intuition so trust you inner guidance on how to meditate.

HOW TO MEDITATE

- Sit in a chair with your feet flat on the floor. Many prefer to sit on the floor in the lotus (cross-legged, with the feet resting on the thighs) or half lotus position.

- Lay your hands with your palms down or up on your lap, or gently clasp hands together.

- Get comfortable, that's most important.

- Ground yourself using the grounding technique we discussed earlier.

- Take in three deep breaths. Relax your mind and body.

- Do not entertain any thoughts that may arise, simply let them pass.

- Keep your attention focused on relaxing and connecting with higher self.

- Meditate for 15-20 minutes daily. You could meditate more or less if you prefer, but establish a routine. Meditate around the same time each day.

****

If you are new to meditation, start off slow. It's better to meditate for 10 minutes each day than one hour a week. You want consistency. You'll find the more you meditate, the more you begin to look forward to the quiet time; the clearer you mind becomes. Establish a routine that works for you. I find

85

meditating first thing in the morning helps to get my day off to a peaceful start.

PRACTICE MEDITATION

Below is a short guided meditation focusing on relaxing your body and connecting with your baby. You may want to read this out loud and record this meditation so you can settle down and listen to it daily.

****

Take in three deep, healing, cleansing breaths. With each breath that you take feel your whole body relaxing. Feel the tension release from each muscle and fiber of your body. Allow your breath to sink deeper within to the very core of your being.

Clear your mind. Let go of anything that has come before this moment. Know that right here and right now is everything. Bring your full attention and awareness to the present. The past has no power, the future is yet to come.

Take your time. Let your mind relax. Let go of all of your thoughts. Trust that in this moment you are being divinely guided and instructed. Listen with your heart. Feel peace and wisdom permeating your very being.

Trust that your body is strong and your baby is healthy. Trust that you are divinely guided and protected. Feel into your body.

Send light to any area that needs support. To send light, simply imagine a bright radiant sun shooting light particles into the top of your head. Allow the light to run through your entire essence. Let this light heal your mind and body. Allow the light to bring you comfort and healing.

Take in another deep breath. Send this breath deep into your body. You have entered a deeper level of awareness.

Now focus your attention on your first chakra, the area between your tail bone and pelvic region. You are going to ground this area to the center of the earth. Pick a grounding cord that feels solid and sturdy to you, something that makes you feel anchored and safe. It can be a big thick rope, or a tree trunk, or even a robust waterfall. Picture it in your mind's eye. Now picture a barbell in the middle of your root chakra. Wrap your grounding cord tightly around the barbell then shoot it down to the center of the earth. Find a huge rock or tree to attach the end of your grounding cord to then pull it tightly. You are now grounded.

Allow this sensation of being grounded to flood your entire being. Relax into it. Breathe into it.

See a golden light running up your grounding cord from the center of the earth. Let this light flood your first chakra. Send the light into every molecule and atom in your pelvic region. Establish a powerful and sacred connection with Mother Earth through your grounding cord.

Now shoot the golden light up through your second, third, fourth, fifth, six and seventh chakras and out the top of your head. Envision this light as a radiant shower engulfing, cleansing and purifying your energy field. Bask in this light and let go of everything else.

Feel clarity coming to you as you ground yourself and cleanse your chakras. Allow your heart to open and soften. Notice how your body feels. Allow relaxation to permeate every cell and fiber of your being. Slow your breathing; feel it become deeper and more rhythmic. Feel yourself becoming lighter energetically.

Say hello to your baby silently. Listen for a voice; pay attention to any pictures, images or impressions you receive in your mind's eye. Your baby may choose to communicate with you in a number of different ways. Take your time. Be attentive!

****

Congratulations! By doing this daily, you will be on your way to establishing intuitive two-way communication with your baby. You've grounded yourself and cleansed and activated your 7 main chakras! After completing the meditation, take a few moments to tune into how you are feeling. Write down your thoughts, feelings, insights and impressions. You are opening up your energy channels and connecting with your intuition and higher self on a sweeter, deeper level. Remember, this is not a race. You get to set your pace. Play with the process and enjoy establishing a partnership with your baby like you've never imagined!

Notes

1. Chopra, Deepak.
   The Chopra Center. *7 Myths Of Meditation* (2016).
   http://www.chopra.com/ccl/7-myths-of-meditation

2. Institute of Noetic Sciences.
   Research. *Meditation Types.* (2016)
   http://www.noetic.org/meditation-bibliography/meditation-types

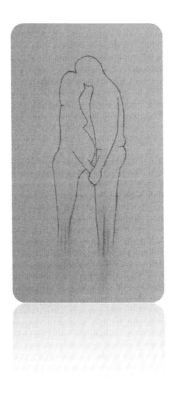

"I am joyfilled and centered.
Divine wisdom guides me."

<u>Notes:</u>

CHAPTER 8
SPECIAL TIPS FOR
YOUR JOURNEY

TOP TEN TIPS

Now that you've learned to ground yourself, meditate, and open your chakras, it's time to be still and go deep within. I've put together my top ten tips to help you develop a deeper spiritual bond with your baby. Keep in mind there is no right or one way to do this. Let your intuition guide you!

    10. *Be gentle and compassionate with yourself.* Love and

honor who you are and your process. Cherish your body temple. Cursing your body adds unnecessary stress and blocks intuition. Cursing the process only pushes away what you truly desire.

9. ***Be open and willing.*** A closed mind and heart will block intuitive communication with your baby. By remaining open and willing, you will be available to hear messages from above and within.

8. ***Meditate regularly.*** Meditation helps you to ground yourself and connect with your intuitive nature. It helps you calm your mind and body.

7. ***Ground yourself frequently.*** Remember a ship in the ocean drops its anchor to be grounded in one place. You ground yourself to bring your own energy back into your space so that you can think clearly and receive divine guidance.

6. ***Keep your chakras open.*** When your chakras are open, energy moves easily, you are able to process information with less effort, and you move fluidly in the world. You need open chakras to communicate with your baby and higher self; to develop your intuition.

5. *Acknowledge your baby as a spiritual being with consciousness and sentience.* We are all spiritual beings having a physical experience. Just like people communicate with loved ones who have passed on, you can communicate with your baby that's coming through. It is a cycle of life—there is no beginning or end to a soul. It is and will continue to be.

4. *Say hello to your baby.* Your baby is excited to talk to you! Say hello and listen for a response. Remember these are intuitive conversations, so pay attention to words or pictures in your head, or feelings. There

is no right or one way to
communicate. Trust yourself.

3. *Practice listening to and
   following your intuition.* It's
   time to go beyond your five
   physical senses and tap into
   your sixth sense, your
   intuition. You have the
   opportunity to receive higher
   levels of information than
   ever before.

2. *Let go of your agenda.* Allow
   your higher self to guide you.
   Step out of your ego. Let go of
   what you think you know or
   think needs to happen and let
   miracles unfold!

1. ***Ask your baby what it needs to be best taken care of in this moment!*** Create a partnership NOW. Intuitive two-way communication opens up infinite channels of possibility between you and your child. You can stop worrying and wondering if you are on track by connecting with your baby and higher self for guidance and instruction.

Enjoy these tips and use them often! Just like the saying goes, "Practice makes perfect," you wouldn't go to the gym once and expect to look like a body builder. The more you use your intuitive muscles, the stronger they will be and the more success you will

100

experience. I know you can do it because I did it. I established intuitive two-way communication with my unborn daughter to navigate my high risk pregnancy. It really works!

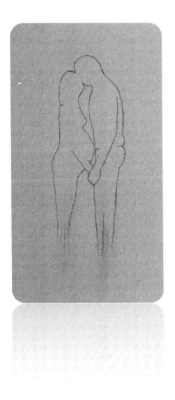

"I lovingly embrace my pregnancy journey."

<u>Notes</u>:

CHAPTER 9

YOUR JOURNEY IS JUST BEGINNING!

THE BEST WAY TO USE THIS BOOK

Wow, you've made it to the end! Rest in the knowledge that you have already opened up the channels of intuitive communication with your baby just by picking up and reading this book. The moment you started reading you sent a divine signal to the universe that you are open and willing to experience a deeper spiritual bond with your baby.

Your little one is listening and waiting to communicate with you!

Think of this book as an instruction manual. Highlight the areas that resonate most with you in this moment, and go back to other parts later. You will notice a difference in the way you feel just by simply practicing one tool in this book! Then work up to practicing more and more tools.

Before I conclude, let's go over a few things again:

- Take time throughout the day to ground yourself. Bringing your energy back into your body will help you feel calmer and more peaceful immediately.

106

- Meditate each morning for 5-15 minutes and notice how grounded you feel during your day.

- Say hello to your baby throughout the day and wait for a response. Your baby may communicate with you with an internal voice you hear in your head, pictures and images, or feelings.

- Practice stretching your intuitive muscles with the exercises outlined in this book, and exercises you create on your own.

- Pay attention. You've opened the door, now expectantly wait for the communication.

That's all for now! If you'd like to dig deeper, I have several videos and articles to support you on your journey. Also, check out my website at SandraJonesKeller.com. I offer personalized Intuitive Pregnancy Coaching and Spiritual Energy Healing sessions tailored to meet your needs. Until next time, happy parenting!

http://sandrajoneskeller.com/

Notes:

Pages to review:

New insights:

Concepts to review:

Made in the USA
San Bernardino, CA
12 August 2020

76985708R00075